CONTENTS

T0020076

to my mother and my father,

for all my midwives

Jordemoder (yoor deh moo' der) – midwife

jord – earth, soil, dust, land, world
moder – mother

—Dictionary of the Swedish Academy, 1934

I. DAUGHTER

The first voice I heard belonged to my mother…
My mother's voice is a lullaby in my cells.

—Terry Tempest Williams, *When Women Were Birds*

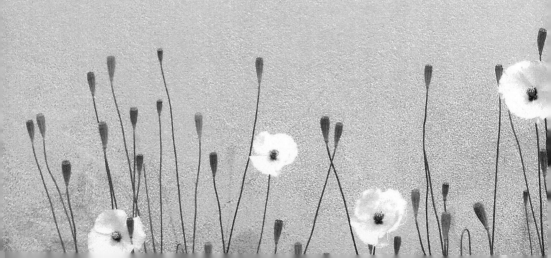

MAW

In the middle of the night, my mother
would bury her face in her
mute, farm-woman's hands
between the hinged high-fidelity
speakers of our Zenith
record player, the soaring
trills of Verdi's dying Violetta
vanquishing the dark.

At the end of the opera,
she'd raise her head, revived,
and I learned from the edge
of the living room: life
turns on passion, as much as breath.

In the middle of the afternoon, I learned
not to be afraid of Virginia Woolf,
Hedda Gabler, Sylvia Plath. And now
when my child goes looking for his mother,
I can explain: it's in the genes,
or a law of nature, or some
all-consuming love—disappearing
into the maw of entropy and art.

AUTODIDACT (FOUND POEM)

The difference between the university graduate and the autodidact lies not so much in the extent of knowledge as in the extent of vitality...
—Milan Kundera

My mother's kitchen table paints an autodidact's life:
books in Swedish, English, German, French,
letters protecting someone's rights,
Nature saved in mass appeals, a mass of daisies
from the yard, a feral cat saved from cold,
day-old coffee she can't discard,
a sketch, a watercolor not yet finished,
like her 8th-grade education—learning
that I can never match.

Today, I find lines on recycled paper:

If I could write poems, I'd write one with questions.
Who makes cranial vises for experiments on cats?
Who makes tasers for goading humans to prison
or animals to slaughter?
Who makes sculpels for cutting
genitals of baby boys?

I sit at my mother's table and sip
reheated coffee, replenishing gall
that graduates lose.

SOMETHING LIKE SALVATION

Whatever is in the world's water is here in my hands.
        —Sandra Steingraber, *Having Faith*

Faithful limbs half-naked before a basin of water, wash rag in hand, my
mother performs her daily ablution. Later, every drop of the graywater will
be re-used to slake her heirloom flowers, or, if the re-cycled rain barrels are
full, to flush her off-the-meter toilet. This morning, she rages at America's
flushing of fire hydrants—well-water pumped from 1000 feet and gushing
like a gashed artery down her gutter—"but I salvaged 50 bucketfuls for
the raspberries!" As I scoop plump berries from Tupperware as old as I am
(derived, she'll tell you, from slag of fossil fuel), I feel the beat of her drum
slow my hand, my tongue, sweeten each jubilant sphere.

MICTURITION GARDENING

The nutrients in urine are in just the right form for plants to drink them up.
    —Håkan Jönsson, researcher of micturition farming,
        Swedish University of Agricultural Sciences, Uppsala

From the bed of her small truck,
my mother brings me her proud wealth:
buckets of ready compost.

Thin skins of allium, dark eyes of tubers,
bitter pits cast from sweet drupes,
guts spilled from beading flesh of melons—

her alchemy of inedibles, her middens
of repeated seasons, turned by her own hand
and catalyzed to gold by a secret ingredient.

She deposits the black buckets at my door
the way a mother bird brings grubs
to her brood or devoted cat drops

a mouse at your feet, proving: the elixir
of love is feeding. My greedy hands
lay it down thick.

SELF-HELP

My mother's arthritic hands grip fistfuls
of green oxalis: heart-leafed weeds she
forages from burgeoning margins
to make my docile chickens go wild.

Spring has a way of pushing up
her dead mother's *You'll never amount to much*
and her dead father's *Another girl....*

From my perch in the kitchen window,
I watch her prop her elbows on the ground,
as clucking hens yank and pluck the tart
hearts, pulsing vitamins.

Once, I heard a midwife say that being unwanted
is more terrible to live with than anything else:
*a child will never get over it.**

But for now, the vying old voices let go
in this animal adoration of survival,
and when all have had their fill, my mother
releases limp remains and pushes herself up.

* Jennifer Worth, *Call the Midwife*

BIRTH DAY

"A birthday should be for a mother
as much as for a child," I say
and kick myself, opening your card.

> Housemaid, waitress, immigrant,
> pregnant with dreams as much as child,
> she was pinned like an insect
> on her back, leather straps
> around her ankles, wrists,
> her mind in the grips
> of an injected amnesiac
> and other women's screams.

I see that you forgot my age this year,
but the faultlines across your falling
face and the familiar fetal fists
say: your body remembers.

> Millimeter by millimeter, fear
> wended down, scarping her inner sacrum,
> buckling her bridge of pubic symphysis,
> rifting her screaming ischial spines
> until, like a god she never believed in,
> the doctor delivered her, and I
> was whisked to another room.
> Nurses bound
> her mammal chest, saying:
> *breastfeeding is barbaric.*

I take up your balled hands
like gifts in mine, unwrap
your still-strong fingers,
unbind your crimped thumbs.

AT THE GREEN BURIAL INFORMATIONAL LUNCHEON

Would I lay my mother's spent stem and flower body
in my bed, intimate with the marriage of love and grief?

Or would I lay her on the kitchen table (pulling out an extra
leaf) where we eat? What will I do with my mother's body

when she is dead? I study the folds of her petal-face
looking forward in the folding chair beside me, and then

the smooth-faced funeral-sellers in front of us, who
seem nice enough, thinking us promising customers.

Her only wish, she states, is to be laid in dirt
less than four feet deep, so the hungry microbes may eat.

"Why does it have to be so complicated, so much paperwork
for the State, rules of custody, transportation—why such fuss?"

No question, I'd prefer to lay her at the foot of the black
walnut tree in my yard, where the strong-willed goldenrod,

tiger lilies and old-world lilacs bloom. I'd want to go there
evenings, recount the news, and how death's ravages

render such feasts of color, pollen, and in spring
the most beloved perfume.

II. MIDWIFE

What else are we to do with our obsessions?
Do they feed us? Or are we simply scavenging our memories
for one gleaming image to tell the truth of what is hunting us?

—Terry Tempest Williams, *When Women Were Birds*

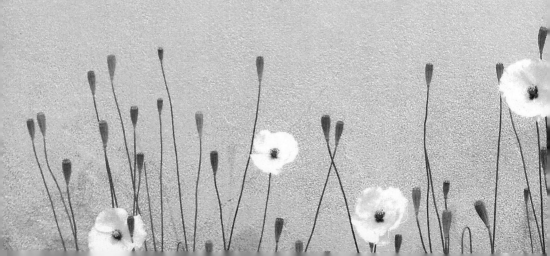

NOVA STELLA

for Lailah

From the out-of-the-blue lull
that can befall hard labor, bestowing
sleep, I could tell

that she was fully dilated
and pronounced her *complete*.
Whereupon she roused, turned

completely dilated eyes to me
and said, with blinding depth and more
love than I have ever seen,

No one ever told me that before,

and reaching down
through a flash and burst
of milky caul
                caught a
                        daughter.

ON BECOMING A MIDWIFE

"What if something happens?"
"You're smart enough to be a doctor."
"Isn't it awfully messy?"
"My births were the best orgasms of my life,"
offered a woman pregnant in the 1970s.

In the beginning, I replied (as a daughter might):
my work is to make mothers happy.

Twenty years on, the 70s mother gone,
a generation of rising
blood pressures, stillbirth, cancer,
even the wild wide-eyed rabbit mother
haunts my door, her perfect child
screaming from the maw
of a righteous lapdog—

I offer words from Mary Oliver:
my work is loving the world.

It is to labor under the name that Linnaeus
gave us: *homo sapiens—wise human,*
and feel a whelm of gratitude for every
caring intelligence: oceans of bodies, bodies
of oceans overwhelmed.

We are mammals, in the end, and my breast
fills with *I can't do this anymore!*, then
ohhh-pen, breeeathe...mi amor! mi amor!

With snapshots, texts: tied tongues,
bleeding nipples, *is an oozing navel normal?*,
baby's first smile, baby's first year...

With poems, poems that plumb
the sweet-salt-metal mess
to climax, over and over, howling *love*.

PHALAENOPSIS

Moth
is what an apostle
of Linnaeus named it.

But at this kitchen table
in this liminal hour, I'm tired
of men's takes on nature.

And Linnaeus, old spy
in your hothouse of flowers,
you might have reconsidered

the tendriled upended genus,
the profane yet prayerful
shape of it, if

just before dawn
you knelt, as a midwife
or a lover does, before

the rising body of a woman:
her epiphytic mind, her
singular surging muscle,

the spreading suspense
of her hips, coming to
a head at tendriled

lips and radiating
Promise.

GRIEF

Tulips of April are too bright
for winter eyes, and the lilac air
steals the breath, suffusing

danger with desire. From my sunlit
kitchen window, I watched a cardinal
proclaim his desire at the top

of the sugar maple—when,
like a heat-seeking missile, he
dropped and trailed a female through air.

How could I not know she would
veer for the glassy glare? I waved my arms
No! as her head hit the double pane

and plain complicities of April killed her.
Penitent for my part, I leave the house
and bear her chilling warmth, heavy

as a stillborn's, to the foot of the maple.
The Cornell lab of ornithology says
every year there are a billion like her.

On my knees in the muddy ground,
I swear I hear the high red buds
in their round oblivion, pull

like a million sapping mouths:
grief is always so much more
than one thing.

THE CYCLE

for Doris—married to a violent, lead-poisoned laborer
and
for Steve—her opiate-addicted son, who murdered Doris,
killed himself, and whose own son died of an overdose

I can gaze for hours at the workings of antlions.
Their conical hollows are like bullet holes
across the sand. Or like little amphitheaters:
whistling pine and twisted juniper for audience.

Their singular feats impressed the fatalist Greeks,
but I am struck by how fragile the traps are—
how easily tragedy can be undone, by
luck of rain or the feet of a happy child.

The antlion is concealed, but I know
that poison is seeping into
his hollow fangs, canny hairs are
quivering along his abdomen—as an ant
going about her ant business, nears
the rim, triggers a grain of sand
and is pulled down. Does she feel
her liquid life seep into the antlion's?
I only see the drained body tossed out.

I am hunted by a Polaroid of us: coffee cups
on a formica kitchen table, he and I
held in the laps of our unhappy mothers.
Later, I was told he hid beneath the bed
when alone with his father,
but all I knew then was: he cried a lot.
I am hunted by questions of

preventability. In the end (or is it the beginning?)
from hunger's wealth of metabolic waste,
beneath the world's abandoned margins,
the antlion spins his rough cocoon, dissolves
and because, as Aristotle said,
nature abhors (but couldn't it be *adores?*)
a vacuum, he is reborn and reborn and re-
born: famished for love and winged
with glistening promise.

SYSTEMIC

The local news repeatedly flashed his steely
black mug like a gun, triggering: fear, hate, hate.

Sad and pathetic that someone births these animals,
wrote a reader of the story in The Washington Times—

a newsfeed that aims to set people like me
right and claims to value: *freedom, faith and family.*

I'd heard enough to question why the media
left out the blamed black mother—that birthing

someone who has a story of repeatedly pleading
for help for her son, when he was in school.

Left out his remembering helpless teacher, racked
with hindsight, with the black-and-white news.

Left out every local black boy pressed against
the barrel of every terrible statistic: stories

swinging forward and backward from the womb.
Left out the local midwife—my ear pressed

to bodies that hold the hearts, the small
parts that right America claims to value,

I hear: *innocent-innocent-innocent.*

VOW

Through her cinched muscular girth,
from stirrups to withers, to her bit
tongue, I could feel the feral
want for the moors of her Baltic island.

On a ride more painful than birth,
the head of my feral right femur
banged against its gnawed pen
of acetabulum, until I asked

myself: what is a horse to humans
but another bearing body to break?
How have I presumed
myself above, unbreakable?

Dismounting and untacking the Russ,
I swore to every Mustang unbroken
in America, to every Brumby unbroken
in Australia, to descendants everywhere

of survivors of conquistadors, wars,
hard labors: *I will not be your breaker.*

THE WIFE WHO MADE A WISH

for Jane

Spring ravished her rooms, bearing musky narcissus and sweet-fleshed
hyacinth blooms. It slipped in through an open window while her husband
was gone, hunting chamois in Switzerland, slipped in with the call of a
cuckoo. Neighbors began to wonder at the abandon everywhere, her hair
coming down and how her blouse-front fell away, the sound of music spilling
out her windows. She wished to be one with everything and set the goats free
to bring life into the place. That is how her husband found her—gamboling
in the garden with a goat—his gun in hand, dried blood of chamois on his
coat. She pulled her blouse together and tried to explain, *the Cuckoo and
Spring,* but a laugh sprang like a shoot from her throat, and as he began to
stammer of scandal and something bestial, *the house stank of something bestial,*
she laughed and laughed until she burst like Spring, into flower.

REPLY

to a mentor

Remember when we waited for the mailman?
Every pen-and-paper letter was an arrival,
every visitor a guest, a reason for making
coffee or something stronger: a drink.
News of death arrived by hand and lips,
and we'd sit together in the living room,
nursing snifters, halting words.

In the subject line on the laptop on my desk,
'Cathy's Passing' stops me dead.
Should I click Reply? Should I Forward?
Should I start a Folder, name it: Cancer?
Can feelings sent through the ether, like
gamma rays through a dissolving brain, help?

I decide to keep it to myself, throw back
a whiskey, hit Delete and write a poem.

TO A GREAT GRANDMOTHER

for Kajsen (1868-1953)

They say you turned
proud with revenge
and bitter as nettles—

untouchable
to God and Men.
I'm writing to tell you:

the gulch in my breast
holds you
and the unborn

children you saved, when
having delivered his 8th
child and watched his

beatings, you refused
to return to the whitewashed
Church for the conjugal

re-purifying: beating
Them at Their
own game.

THE WAY ART LIVES

I see the small lives
lost in the making
of your luminous
silk scarf, smooth
and soft as newborn
skin, its spun protein
fibers finer than hair.
It contains you
the way a cocoon
contains metamorphosis,
the way the pia mater
contains memory,
the way the amnion
in your loomed womb
contained a spinning son.

THE APPRENTICE BECOMES A MIDWIFE

for Miranda

The apprentice puts his body where the body of the teacher is.
                —Garrett Hongo, as quoted by apprentice/poet Jesse Bertron

With the apprentice's catch
of breath, I register the purpling head,
the turtled neck—a shoulder stuck
on a bridge of bone.

Exhaling as one, we become
four hands at a piano,
playing a difficult fugue.
This time, her embodied
measures lead mine:

roll to hands and knees now;
please over to your back again;
now over again, one knee up
and push....

Your baby's born!
Feel free to welcome her,
we're giving her
a few breaths, the cord
is giving her oxygen—

the newborn cries,
the mother raises her up
and—paused on the bridge
to separation—the wet
eyes of the apprentice
meet my own.

IMAGINE YOU ARE A MIDWIFE

Sometimes, the most you can do
said Lao-Tzu, some 2000 years ago, is

imagine you are a midwife.
Do good without show or fuss.

When the baby is born, the mother
may say: I did it! I am equal to life!

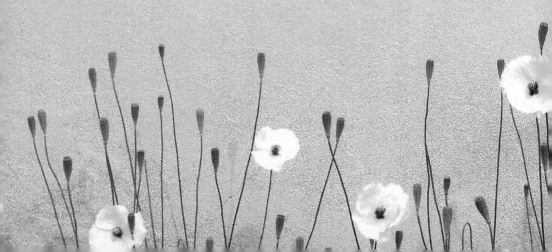

III. MOTHER

If a child is to keep alive his inborn sense of wonder,
he needs the companionship of at least one adult who
can share it....

—Rachel Carson, *The Sense of Wonder*

HATCHLINGS

Breastfeeding on the porch, I listen
to a chorus of hooligan hatchlings
erupt whenever food appears: *me, me, me!*

The greed of summer takes me back
to an American soccer player who ran at
the ball, muttering: *get it, get it, get it!*

Then, to a stork-like Swiss man who
pulled off my shoe, as the train pulled out
and tucking his strange love under his arm,
leaped onto the vanishing platform.

Then to Paris: perfumed Moroccan men
swooping around me and my au pair friends
like swifts along the Seine, hunting supper.

And in fairness, to myself at eighteen, when
I chased an older man to the Cotswolds.
We lay beside the River Leach
and small round bells, attached to shins
of ribald Morris dancers, jangled
in the distance, just

like baby birds in Wisconsin,
bobbing up and down in hunger.

TO RAISE A SON

The hens have started laying again.
So, with renewed
eagerness, this Easter morning,
my young son and I
clean the chicken coop
(*fowls' foul* nests, we joke)
and sift rabbit poop
from the chicken food.
I tell him about Eostre,
goddess of spring, who
(stories say) saved a bird
with frozen wings by transforming
her into an egg-laying rabbit.
"Why?" he likes to ask.
"For luck," I guess, "perhaps
in overcoming death,"
and that makes me bring up the dark
ages, when ever-hedging humans
began to color eggs like
flowers, like jewels
holding precious suns.
"That's what we'll be doing," he
adds, as we chat with each
hen by name and ponder
the meaning of her calls, then
free their dinosaur bodies
to run and scratch and sprawl
in sunny oases of sand.
"Do you think that dinosaurs
loved our sun this much?" I ask.
"More, if they were cold-blooded,"
he reasons, knowing
some argue they were not,
and at last, we open the laying
box: "Four eggs!" he shouts,
bloomed and warm.

RUSH HOUR

A pterosaur, my son might call him—
the 10-million-year-old sandhill crane
in flight above 8 lanes of traffic.

Suddenly, my morning soars with
hope, gratitude: may he continue

to ride the thermals after all the tar
sands have been extracted, after
all the fossils have flown.

NEIGHBORHOOD VIOLENCE THAT NOBODY TALKS ABOUT
(as I drive my son to school one rainy morning)

Streets as wide as airport strips.
Sidewalks never laid.
Cars at stop signs over-running zebra stripes.
Pedestrians scattering like prey.
My son's locked school.
No Guns Allowed (a sign on his way into 5th grade).
Continuing on, by weedless playgrounds, weedless lawns,
a golf course beside an unswimmable city lake.
The ghost-white bicycle where a child was killed.
A Starbuck's barista: *Have a nice day!*
Another flooding rain.

FEELING GAME

Before dying, explains the child I birthed,
you become critical. When critical, you're prone,
with loud breathing and disorienting effects.

      Okay, I say over his shoulder, feeling game,
      that's how your uncle was, before going sober,
      how mothers are in hard labor, and how
      I become, listening too much to the news.

He rolls his eyes at his mother's *personalizing* everything
and says, I'm talking about stamina: low stamina prevents
action, sprints, melees. I need more experience.

      Okay, I say, strong in experience, I get it:
      you level up from the pain, or dark spirits,
      then fight like a mother for better gun control—
      is that the point of video-gaming?

TAKING MY YOUNG COFFEE-DRINKER TO THE OLD CAFE

We step into the place where the old
cafe had been, glassy now and spacious,
silent with down-turned faces,
crimped necks and thumbs.

Where has the carnival of coffee gone?
Real Italian baristas, flashing levers
and espresso eyes? I used to imbibe
every delectable detail of them—large men

embodying their grind: strong black brows
and oxen necks, slung in aprons of fresh white.
I hear their echoing operatic vowels:
Un caffè! Caffè latte! Cappucino!

I was the loner in the corner, who needed
a place to write, while the old regulars
needed a place to walk their dogs to
mornings, and young people

got taught the fine slow art of froth.

FIRST DAY

I've watched his life layers build up
and the warm mother sea recede.

He towers now, taller than I am.
I know that life goes in stages and high school

is just another beginning, but beholding
him today, I see the moist newborn skin, his first

furrow of eyebrows and easily could sink again
into our family bed. As he snaps his bike helmet

into place and squints up the sunlit street into
his future, mothers everywhere hold back

their tidal nature, and I wave *goodbye*
as naturally, he speeds off.

FALL HEAT

From the wide kitchen window,
I watch the aging speckled hen scratch
with a mother's vigor against a slanting sun,
as late mote-filled rays smolder her umber
feathers and spotlight the compost bin
in the corner—summer's last cauldron of heat.

I feel that by writing, I am doing what is
far more necessary than anything else,
wrote Virginia Woolf, in what would prove
the late autumn of her life.

In the birdbath, starlings close their roiling show
while ruly cedar waxwings sit in the cedar tree
and wait their turn. Notwithstanding my patient
husband, pruning perennials, seeding balding
patches of lawn, I let supper wait, grab
a pen and stir my compost-heart.

WINTER SOUP

You might be chopping beets
listening to public radio reports
on political gerrymandering,
presidential sex scandals,
the latest mass shooting or proof
of global warming, when you
glance out your steamed-up kitchen
window and see a boy down the block
bound out of his mother's house and clear
a thawing lawn in three leaps, as a girl
in sturdy boots steps off of a bus.

Looking forward, the way nurses
instruct convalescents to find their feet,
she commandeers the slippery street
and walks into his naked, open arms.

Is it the boy's transparent love, so like
your son's? Or is it the reassuring fact—
despite robins too early on your lawn—
that she seems so much readier for life
than you were then, that makes you
turn the radio off and tune your whole
heart to the crimson globes at hand?

TO MY SON, GRADUATING

Our house is on fire.
          —Greta Thunberg, youth climate activist

Together, beneath sweet Scheherezade lilies,
I mull over one-thousand-and-one
nights of labor—stories
that by degrees, made a warp, a weft,
a safety net, a parachute in the life
I've been lucky enough to weave.
Beside us, beneath a merciful
morning sun, two deaf old hounds
with cataracts and sundown syndrome.

It was never enough
to make the world safer for you, my
Greta-aged, graduating son—by all means,
take a gap year! Keep your hair long,
sing out loud to all the good songs:
burn the house down. And if only
to assuage your mother, stop
to smell the flowers, imprint
their perfume as we head
into immeasurable, untold crises.

IV. INVANDRARE

Swedish word for 'immigrant';
literally, 'in-wanderer'

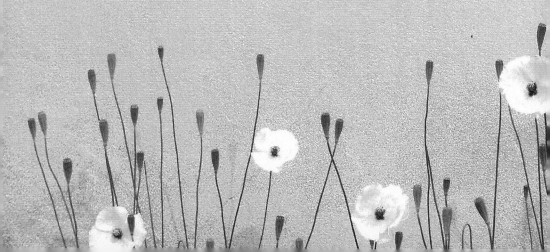

STILL LIFE

Cardamom buns baked on parchment,
percolated coffee in thin-lipped cups,
a porcelain pitcher of cream,
and reflecting a south Chicago
sun, a crystal pyramid
of sugar cubes, silver-plated tongs.
On our way to the guests,
my mother would say in Swedish,
Be nice and take that one, and I knew
the bun she meant: the least lovely one.
I loved her no less—her gold plaited
hair and cerulean blue eyes,
like a hand-painted doll
made not for play but to please.

Here I am, fifty-three,
in an old-world *konditori*
and might as well be ten—aswirl
with cardamom, and catching my breath
at a glinting plate of sugar cubes,
an elegant pitcher of cream.
"Hej!" greets a Swedish young man
at the counter, startling me out of my past.
I smile back and point
to the loveliest bun I see, pour
self-serve coffee into an Ikea cup
and sit at a table with a real cloth,
as if all the dolls grew up
and left a still-beloved house.
I want for nothing, but my mother
sitting with me.

THIN PLACES

The dogs and I lift our heads and sniff the air,
the way infants catch their first breaths, curling

back their necks and open to being mammal.
The old limestone city is blanketed in snow,

but our noses lead us toward something
warm, steamy, slightly sweet, when

our ears perk up—a call? a whistle?
Our senses pull us down the street

and lift our gaze to a gable window,
like a beacon in the northern night.

My Lutheran grandmother warned me
not to take after my mother, forever

losing herself in time. Not to be
like the ruminating sheep, grazing

among the cairns. But the window is open
and a trill pours out the way joy pours out

the bright yellow mouth of a blackbird!
The dogs and I stand patient as statues

as aromas of Swedish pancakes drift down.
Then, she leans out—a flushed young woman

damp from the heat of the skillet and fanning
her neck with a towel, swirls of wet curls

spilling out a bright yellow scarf.
And just as suddenly, she's gone.

But the air remains almost edible,
and her trills keep falling like stars.

SWEDISH PANCAKES

should be tawny gold in color, from yellow fat
of whole milk from brown cows in pasture
and yolks like suns from farmyard hens;

should be soft as satin, yet latticed at the edges
from batter poured into a satisfied skillet
riding tides of butter to caramel rims;

are richest made from colostrum, first sweet milk
at calving time, when everyone on the farm
rides tides of common good.

OUT AMONG THE GRASS AND THISTLES

cows graze between the rune stones, raised
to honor noble deeds, making milk.

Even the white chickens, upon whom so much
also depends, embody importance and dwarf
my daily laying of vowels, consonants,

churnings of a scavenging mind.
As if feeding a hunger I can't control, I toil
every waking hour and even half-asleep

to crack the mystery of gravel in a crop
grinding grain, grubs, insects,
dust into something noble and whole.

MAIEUTIC

from the Greek, maieutikos: "to act as a midwife;"
the name that Socrates gave his method of inquiry
with the aim of bringing forth implicit understandings

Seated near the cafe window
a woman stares at the sea and sways.
She stays this way for two hours.
Illness? Prayer?
The quivering of her hijab
suggests: weeping.

Turning spent eyes on me, she asks,
what is the cost to leave this island?

I believe she's mistaken me
for a local with wealth
or answers for everything,
then I see that she's pregnant:
instinct tells her that I, too
am an outsider, swollen with turmoil.

Is this what my grandmother meant
when she muttered, *it's hard to be human?*

Sooner or later, everybody's buffeted
to the margins in pregnancy, marriage,
war—all the mergings and expulsions
that we are made in, die in,
risk unknown borders for.

I tell her, I don't know
what it costs to leave the island
but lean toward her and ask
if she would like to walk together
to the budding harbor.

We sway beneath the quivering
calyxes of May, braving crisis.

SABBATICAL IN A SWEDISH HANSEATIC CITY

Narrative is radical, creating us at the very moment it is being created.
            —Toni Morrison

Open, deep-welled windows
of our rented 17th-century house
home, like ears, to hourly bells
of a medieval cathedral and to
luggage wheels, clapping like
applause across the hand-hewn cobbles.

In the bed, the snores of my husband
sound like bombs being dropped.
When the dread siren rises from passages
inside his head, I used to shrink beneath
the covers, but now I hold his hand:
this can quiet the implosions.

If the siren starts again, I sit up—this
is when I'm awake the tolling hours, listening
past the walls and marveling over
how far we've come, despite divided
countries, our disavowed perfect union.

Some nights, my husband purrs.
Purring is called *spinning* here. His gentle
whir secures my sleep and turns the insides
of my eyelids orange and pink, like petals
of roses that climb the houses along
our street like dreams—this is when
I wake with the sun and the cooing
of a dozen doves: who was it

who said, whoever tells the best story wins?
At the window, I see their stained-
glass breasts: jewels set in a World
Heritage wall that rings our middle-ages
town like a shimmering league of nations,
like radical ramparts of peace!

RUINS

Visiting Americans ask me, why
are there public drunks in Sweden?

Like the intelligent jackdaws
my son is named after, alcohlics flock
from public housing to morning benches
preened and eager, filled with laughter.
By afternoon, they slump and stagger—
haggard with forgetting and sorrow.

I don't know, I used to answer, *the Nordic climate?*

It disgusts the tourists to see them
urinate against the UNESCO-protected
Hanseatic wall, built by wealthy men
for war against peasants: ruins
are supposed to be pretty.

But the sun, like a god in the North,
will shine again on a bench
in the morning and make everything
seem possible—a cycle I can relate to—
and now, when Americans ask me, I try

to explain: *the public, the sun, the Nordic Model.*

STOCKHOLM PUBLIC ART

Sweden ranks as the world's happiest country for women,
as self-reported in public surveys of human rights, gender
equality, income equality, progress and safety.
                    —U.S. News & World Report, 2021

Two concrete sows, large as life and smiling
with contentment—their realistic teats
mountainous with milk and piglets.

Alongside the un-named public art, a litter of toddlers
squeals and scrambles up a set of playground bars,
suggesting, *Bars Are Meant for Climbing,*

while across the top of the sprawled flanks
of the free-range sows, two human mothers sit down
and put their feet up, suggesting, *Happy Mothers—*

when, opening their blouses and lifting eager infants
to filling breasts, they raise their smiling faces to the sun
and crown the art: *A Pinnacle of Culture.*

PARADE TO THE GRADUATION BALL

Typically, classic cars
are not my thing—top-down
Eldorados, Mustangs, Firebirds
and behind the wheels: classic men.

But I'm transfixed by the bare young
women in the seats behind them—
graduates, stiff as statues in competing
decolletages and blue as scilla
in the Baltic spring, and beside them:
fully clothed young men.

Except for the cars, the old town square
could be a painting by some Old
Master—I swear, the more things change
the more things stay the same.

Then a murmur goes up, and I see
a wide-fendered bicycle, wheeled
by a wild-maned young woman
in confident heels and a high-necked
fiery gown, and the town

erupts in cheers! If I were some old
Breughel, I'd paint the whole
spectacular thing.

IT TAKES A DOG

A fellow foreigner plods toward
my outdoor cafe table and kneels
before my two wagging dogs.

Leaning forward in his ten-gallon
hat, snakeskin boots and gold
filigree buckle, he whispers to them.

I watch as their pink eager tongues
brighten him. Raising himself up,
he winks at me, then drawls:

"Sometahmes it takes a dawg
to make the world raht agin,"
and leaves—before I can reach

out and catch the Lone Star,
before I can tell him in eager
English, *I understand you!*

THE INGMAR BERGMAN SAFARI

There is no country where the incomprehensible
is more cherished, than in Sweden.
        —Theodor Kallifatides, *Ett nytt land utanför mitt fönster*
        (*A new land outside my window*)

Who spends a summer day in Sweden going on an Ingmar Bergman safari, instead of going to the beach, or the French creperie up the road?

I board the bus, spot an unclaimed seat at the back and slide past a woman from Portland calling herself an *existential feminist* and saying, "I dig Bergman's women, man," then Swedes blaming Norwegians for claiming seats that the Swedes had claimed for friends, and land beside a wordless man in glasses.

A straight-shooting sheep farmer stands up, shushes us and introduces herself as tour director. She assures us, as promised in the brochure, that we'll stop at all the sites of films made on Fårö: Sheep Island.

The bus drives first to the lonely coast where *Persona* was filmed, while screens above our heads play scenes from the film that reflect the scenery outside. It is a story of two women: Alma, chatty and carefree, and Elisabet, an actress, mute and in exile from the staged world, in pursuit of her buried self.

Meanwhile, across the aisle, a voluptuous Brazilian is being played by a Frenchman seated beside his writing wife. The wife reminds me of Elisabet and words by Marguerite Duras: *Ecrire, c'est aussi ne pas parler. C'est hurler sans bruit.* Writing is also not to speak. It is to howl noiselessly.

Maybe it's true. All the world's a stage, and all of us are players, sitting in different life ages, playing our inexorable parts.

Next, the bus pulls up beside the house of Bergman's ex-wife, where *Scenes from a Marriage* was shot. The screens play the part where a professor tells his wife that he's leaving her for a younger woman and Paris—a scene, our director informs us, straight from Bergman's life. *Where we stand and bleat about our loneliness without listening to each other...stare into each other's eyes and yet deny each other's existence.* The wives, she adds, turned out happier.

And so the safari goes, tracking human highs and lows: *The Passion of Anna* and *Shame*. As the sun descends toward the Baltic in the west, the tour draws to a close over a grilled lamb picnic. We eat facing the sun, on the coast where *Through a Glass Darkly* was filmed about descending into schizophrenia. I ruminate on my brother, my grandmother.

Returning to the lot where the tour began, like a finale, our shepherd-director plays one film more: Bergman's homage to his island neighbor, a fisherman married to the sea. The eternal plots play out: a day dawning, seagulls crying, insects hunting and being hunted, oars revolving in their locks—the herring, the hauling, the mooring, the making of fire in a stove—the world concluding its night's fast. Throughout, the fisherman moves as one, plays only himself.

I look around the quiet bus and wonder: is this the part that our far-flung lives were after? Like a satisfied return from a hunt?

Or is it more like a dawning and a cherishing of everything in front of us? Around us. In us. Home. Maybe it's the cry of the artist for re-claiming, for re-pairing a human life.

Two rows down, I see the Portlandian has landed a professor.

ODE TO A PUBLIC LIBRARY

Paradise will be a kind of library.
                    —Jorge Luis Borges

This afternoon, a Masai-boned Estonian is singing runes.
The translucent leaves of her eyelids close, and her willowy

white arms leap, as if tracing words in stone, living letters
from the dead. Her body is a song of thousand-year-old

harvests, losses, loves and a sympathetic drone
from deep within her breast thrums through mine.

We sit in the front row, my son and I, embraced by
multi-storied stacks and windows, vistas of our fairytale

city and sea beyond, serrated like steel beneath
a winter sun, the white caps of Aegir's daughters waving.

Here we are millionaires in second-hand clothes: he sips
hot cocoa, and I sip bottomless coffee for 20 crowns.

I think of our public library as a kind of paradise, a kind
of democracy on earth, where the ancient and the recent

and the soon dead meet and open like doors
to hunger, abundance, wonder, grief. Next week,

balalaikas will sing their hearts out in strings,
with violins and accordions entering in

like some gathering force of arms for peace with Russia.

WINTER RENOVATIONS AT THE CLARION

Tourists flock. Even the luxury hotel
windows peer with prurient eyes, down
on the two unknowns: the human bones
being exposed, separated, unhomed.

I think of my aging parents, poring
over obituaries, the way cluing bones
cue the curious flesh to sing—
a local pastor sounds a cry of protest,

while scientists say the female
is about seventeen, that she
and the child within her arms
are pre-Christian, no tourists here.

For my part, I imagine they belong
to the stock of farming and fishing folk
on the island and spoke their sea-sun-earth
language. That they belong to the spiral-
horned sheep, hefted to this Silurian rock,
and to the hefty horses, their thick manes

and coats. We mull in our thinsulate
jackets, relish the curling breath
on our lips, as if proof
of a higher existence, yet

we vie to peer into the pit, to grasp
their embrace of mineral and humus.

RAUKS

columns of fossilized rock, formed as softer
geological material is eroded away; from Gutnish,
a language native to the island of Gotland

Born in warm, embryonic seas,
the crusty giants
once were pulsing
nerve centers, teeming coral.
Earth's own cranium shifted
them from their biogenous beds.
Gnarled and knobbly with life
and death, they stand today
along a Baltic coast exposing
their naked hearts—
earth's best poems!
Or brainstems,
freed from
softer matter.
I like to go
and dangle
my knobby
feet below
one—
midbrain,
pons,
medulla
oblongata—
feeling
happy.

V. HOME

*A great longing is upon us, to live again
in a world made of gifts.*

—Robin Wall Kimmerer, *Braiding Sweetgrass*

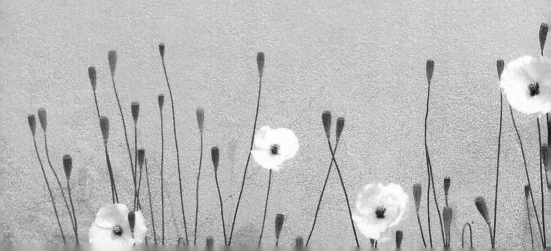

IN THE BOTANICAL GARDENS

A sun-drenched bed
of snowdrops and winter aconite,

white-tailed bumblebees, even pigeons
beckon to me, strutting iridescent breasts

and looking me sideways in the eye.
Spring's first polished motorcycle rumbles by

but can't compete with a wren's tremble-chatter
or this ancient magnolia, pink galleon

acrest a sea of yellow-white.
I linger amidst her silver limbs.

A woman who reminds me of someone
sails by, a weathered book in her weathered

hands, in her smiling eyes: mine.
Love after fifty is like love before

the age of five, unable to contain itself.
Now, I'm the unconditional bench;

now, the magnificent tree; now
the whispering sweet air, and petals

like kisses rain through me.

VITAL SIGNS

Crocuses still open
their saffron hearts.

And noiseless
pink opossum feet

land like cherry blossoms
beneath the suet feeder.

As they've always done,
velvet-nosed lambs, tails

twirling, thrust and suckle
their sure-footed moms.

And cows with calves gallop out
stale winter barns and jump

for joy, kicking their Eocene heels
impossibly high—

the tumbling udders
shuddering anybody with joy

and signaling *Spring*
on a thriving family farm.

SUNDAYS WITH MY FATHER

"My fault, Guv'nor!" An East London
skateboarder vaulted from the walk

and apologized to my father.
That family vacation was the first

time I heard that a fault was not
my father's. These days, after his stroke,

glaucoma, heart surgery, a pacemaker,
we reminisce over apple pie and ice cream

or his favorite: French toast (*lost bread*,
in French, I tell him—he relishes frugality).

We speak of his mother's schizophrenia:
painful boyhood trips to the 'mental institution.'

After high school, his job in the Loop:
scrimping and saving for a home, a happy

wife, his children's education. The time he
crawled from his sickbed, evading death

to complete the taxes. Marching for love
and peace through Vietnam, Civil Rights,

the Cold War, a nuclear arms race, divorce,
his son's psychosis. This week, I'll tell him

it was never lost on us: his perfect love
for our nuclear family.

MUSE

Hurrying home in heavy snowfall,
I'm stopped in my tracks
by the *hoo-h' Hoo-hoo-hoo*
of a great horned owl.

Tempted to turn from the trampled
sidewalk into the snowy wood
and find him, I call instead
to a hooded stranger across the street:

Did you hear that gorgeous male owl?
The stranger doesn't look up—
earbuds maybe, or assumes I'm crazy.
Anyway, what would I do if

I found him? The haunting hunter
who helped me hear a calling
greater than men must be long married
by now, an empty-nester. Still,

he turns my head and sounds my animal heart.

MAINTENANCE MAN

Computer maintenance was not among
my criteria for a husband, father of my child.

Back then, who could have imagined
the life-or-death, love-and-hate

necessity of a screen?
I still don't know what it means:

computer maintenance.
Then again, he doesn't really know

what it means to write poems.
So, imagine how I swooned

when I googled a thing he does:
defragmenting—

a process of locating small parts
and rearranging them into a whole.

It made me go and fling
my arms around him, my

maintenance man—transforming
file into *life*—my poet by another name!

END TIMES

Today, Death Valley
nearly topped the hottest
recorded temperature on earth.
Here in the Midwest, we
breathe the smoke from Canada.
The roses (cultivars) are perishing
in the heat. Resistant tiger lilies
stand a chance, if rabbits
(toppling stems to strip the leaves)
and chipmunks (chomping
buds like cobs of corn) are
somehow checked.

A friend, checked by life in recent years,
texts: Jesus has been speaking to me.
He said, 'Tell the world I'm coming!'

I believe we have this in common:
a dream of escape from the late
Anthropocene. But in terms
of space travel, I text back:
I'll stay here. In time of Rapture,
I'll go to the bed of *Aesclepias*—
milkweed, snaking underground
and send up complex mixed-sex flowers,
then pods of silver-haired seeds
that will sail prevailing winds
to a new age of monarchs, of
multiplying hymenoptera.

HOPE

for Hannu

At the birth of a third daughter
on the eve of World War,
my grandfather refused to look
at her, or come in from the barn.
In that old country, deep
within my newborn mother
in my invisible ovary home,
I must have learned: hope
is complicated.

Did my someday-son learn it too,
when the New World obstetrician
strapped my immigrant mother
down, told her *shut up*,
cut the pulsing umbilical cord
and slapped me into air?
America was in Vietnam, wars at home,
Silent Spring took the world
by storm and soon, I was marching
for peace in the arms of a loving father.
I must have learned: hope
is not for the fainthearted.

The summer I turned fifty
and my child became a teen, wildfires
burned where they never burned before,
schools were locked down, seas
were heating up, crops were under
water, waves of children flooded
borders as if to cry: hope
demands looking!

We watch from the swing now, you and I,
below the spiraling trumpet vine
in the garden, planted by you the year
our son was born in the bed upstairs.
A fanfare of open-throated flowers
sweetens the return
of ruby-throated hummingbirds: *hope*
is the thing with feathers—[*]
stubborn birds, small as ovaries,
defying sore odds
for nectar.

* Emily Dickinson, *"Hope" is the thing with feathers*

ACKNOWLEDGMENTS

I am grateful to the following publications in which some of the poems first appeared, often in provisional form or with a different title:

Ars Medica: A Journal of Medicine, The Arts, and Humanities: "Grief," "Imagine You Are a Midwife," "The Way Art Lives"

Eastern Iowa Review: "Something Like Salvation," "The Wife Who Made a Wish" (winner of Editor's Choice award and nominated for Best of the Net)

Intima: A Journal of Narrative Medicine: "At the Green Burial Informational Luncheon" (nominated for a Pushcart Prize)

Midwest Review: "Maw," "Out Among the Grass and Thistles"

Minerva Rising: "Autodidact (found poem)"

Mom Egg Review: "Nova Stella," "Phalaenopsis"

Plant-Human Quarterly: "In the Botanical Gardens," "Phalaenopsis"

Wisconsin Fellowship of Poets Calendar: "Swedish Pancakes"

Wisconsin People & Ideas: "Hope" (nominated for a Pushcart Prize), "Still Life"

Thanks to all the families who have honored me with their trust. Thanks to Robin Chapman, Katsi Cook, Marge Piercy, Andrea Potos, Cherene Sherrard, Enid Shomer and Juliana Spahr for, amidst their own pressing labors, making time for my first book. Thanks to Samuli Jortikka for sharing his enticing cover photograph from Gotland, where this book was conceived. Thank you, Gotland. My gratitude to Lailah Shima, Miranda Welch and Catherine Young for years of support and encouragement, as well as for dedicated reading and commenting. I cannot count, or thank enough, Miranda's focused hours. Boundless gratitude to Karolina Johnson, Alfred Johnson and Karl Johnson for lifelong love and generosity; they made this book possible. To Hannu and Kai: my love and gratitude forever for seeing me (us) through.

ABOUT THE AUTHOR

INGRID ANDERSSON has practiced as a home-birth nurse midwife for over 20 years. She studied poetry and literature in Swedish, German, French and English, as well as anthropology, at the University of Wisconsin-Madison, before mixing that fertile ground with the art and science of midwifery (Frontier Nursing University, 2000). Ingrid is a healthcare activist and founder of related nonprofits. Her poetry has been nominated for a Pushcart Prize and Best of the Net and has appeared in *Ars Medica, Eastern Iowa Review, Midwest Review, Minerva Rising, Plant-Human Quarterly* and elsewhere. She lives in Madison, Wisconsin with her Swedish-Finnish husband, son, dogs, chickens and bees. *Jordemoder* is her debut collection.

For more information, please visit *www.www.ingridandersson.info*